Review of

Diabetes Mellitus

In

Pregnancy

AUTHOR

DR.ANKUSH NANDKISHOR RAUT

Everyday new recommendations and guidelines coming for diabetes in pregnancy. This book will acknowledge you about screening, diagnosis, complications and management of diabetes in pregnancy. Will definitely help you to solve questions related to diabetes in pregnancy in MRCOG examination.

Preface:

Approximately 700,000 women give birth in England and Wales each year, and up to 5% of these women have either pre-existing diabetes or gestational diabetes. Women who have diabetes during pregnancy, it is estimated that approximately 87.5% have gestational diabetes (which may or may not resolve after pregnancy), 7.5% have type1 diabetes and the remaining 5% have type 2 diabetes. Diabetes affect both women as well as fetus. There is increase in risk of abortion, malformation, preterm labour, gestational hypertension, macrosomia, shoulder dystocia and sudden infant death in women with diabetes in pregnancy. There is lots of controversies regarding screening programme and management. Recently HAPO study come up with new guidelines for diagnosis of gestational diabetes mellitus. HAPO study also study various effect of diabetes on fetus and mother. Accordingly national institute for health and care excellence update guideline for diabetes in pregnancy which give us clear idea about screening and management. This book will help you to understand screening for diabetes, diagnostic criteria, effect of diabetes on mother , effect of diabetes on fetus, management of overt and gestational diabetes mellitus. Hope review will help you to manage pregnancy with diabetes more effectively.

Index:

<u>DEDICATION</u>

To all students of Obstetrics & Gynaecology and my family who light up my life.

To my wife Sonali who has been there for me from the beginning.

Introduction

Prevalence in less than 30 age group is 5.4%. Of women who have diabetes during pregnancy, it is estimated that approximately 87.5% have gestational diabetes (which may or may not resolve after pregnancy), 7.5% have type1 diabetes and the remaining 5% have type2 diabetes. The prevalence of type1 diabetes, and especially type2 diabetes, has increased in recent years. The incidence of gestational diabetes is also increasing as a result of higher rates of obesity in the general population and more pregnancies in older women.

Classification:

a) Type 1 diabetes
b) Type 2 diabetes
c) other specific types:
   a. Genetic defects of beta cell function
   b. Genetic defects in insulin function
   c. Disease of the exocrine pancreas (pancreatitis, neoplasia, hemochromatosis)
   d. Endocrinopathies (Acromegaly, Cushing`s syndrome, Pheochromocytoma.)
   e. Drug or chemical induced (glucocorticoids and thiazides, beta adrenergic agonist)
   f. Infections (congenital rubella, cytomegalovirus)
   g. Uncommon forms of immune mediated diabetes
   h. Other genetic syndrome (Down`s syndrome, Klinfelter`s syndrome, Turner`s syndrome)
d) Gestational diabetes mellitus

Type 1 diabetes:

➢ Insulin dependent or juvenile onset diabetes mellitus.
➢ Manifests at childhood or adolescent period.
➢ Requires exogenous insulin.
➢ Because of autoimmune destruction of pancreatic beta cell.
➢ Hashimoto`s thyroiditis, Graves' disease, Addison`s disease, vitiligo, celiac sprue, autoimmune hepatitis, myasthenia gravis, and pernicious anaemia associated with it.

> ➢ HLA on chromosome 6 is responsible, but vertical transmission is low and concordance rate for twin is less than 50%.
> ➢ But small proportion of type 1 diabetics, mostly Africans and Asians, lack evidences for autoimmunity and not associated with HLA, but show strong inheritance.

Type 2 diabetes mellitus:

> ➢ Account for 90 to 95% of diabetes.
> ➢ Non-insulin dependent or maturity onset.
> ➢ No beta cell destruction but insulin produce is insufficient or insulin resistance. So relative deficiency. Hyperglycaemia may exist several years prior to identification.
> ➢ Obesity important factor for insulin resistance. Although no HLA association but 100% concurrence for monozygotic twins. Women with gestational diabetes mellitus have greater chances of development of type 2 diabetes in future.

Gestational diabetes mellitus:

> ➢ Prevalence: 1 to 14%

"Any degree of glucose intolerance with onset or first recognition during pregnancy."

Approximately 700,000 women give birth in England and Wales each year, and up to 5% of these women have either pre-existing diabetes or gestational diabetes. Women who have diabetes during pregnancy, it is estimated that approximately 87.5% have gestational diabetes (which may or may not resolve after pregnancy), 7.5% have type1 diabetes and the remaining 5% have type2 diabetes. The prevalence of type1 diabetes, and especially type2 diabetes, has increased in recent years. The incidence of gestational diabetes is also increasing as a result of higher rates of obesity in the general population and more pregnancies in older women.

Divided into:

a) Pre-gestational or overt
b) Gestational diabetes

Table 1: White's classification in pregnancy:

Class	Onset	Fasting	2 Hour post prandial	Therapy
A1	Gestational	<105mg/dl	<120mg/dl	Diet
A2	Gestational	>105mg/dl	>120mg/dl	Insulin
Class	Age of onset	Duration	Vascular disease	Therapy
B	Over 20	<10	None	Insulin
C	10 to 19	10 to 19	None	Insulin
D	Before 10	>20	Benign retinopathy*	Insulin
F	Any	Any	Nephropathy	Insulin
R	Any	Any	Proliferative retinopathy	Insulin
H	Any	Any	Heart	Insulin

All above values indicate plasma glucose levels. *Nephropathy when diagnosed during pregnancy: Proteinuria greater than or equals to 500mg/24 hour before 20 weeks gestation.

White classification is no longer recommended now, instead focus is on whether diabetes antedates pregnancy or is first diagnosed during pregnancy so new classification proposed by ADA is:

Table 2

Gestational diabetes:	Diabetes diagnosed during pregnancy that is not clearly overt (type 1 or type2) diabetes.
Type 1	**Type 2**
Diabetes resulting from beta cell destruction, usually leading to absolute deficiency a) Without vascular complications b) With vascular complications	Diabetes from inadequate insulin secretion in the face of increase insulin resistance a) Without vascular complications b) With vascular complications
Other type of diabetes: Genetic in origin, drug induced, chemically induced	

Pre-gestational (overt diabetes):

Diagnosis:

Women with high plasma glucose level >200mg/dl (with or without classical signs of polyuria, polydipsia and unexplained weight loss), glycosuria, ketoacidosis prior to pregnancy.

If women come do not have history of DM then diagnosis is done by IADPSG criteria:

Table 3:

Diagnosis of overt diabetes during pregnancy:	
Measure of glycaemia	Threshold
Fasting plasma glucose	At least 7.0 mmol/L (126 mg/dl)
HBA1c	At least 6.5%
Random blood glucose	At least 11 mmol/L (200 mg/dl)

Apply to women without known diabetes antedating pregnancy. The decision to perform blood testing for evaluation of glycaemia on all pregnant women or women with characteristics of indicating a high risk for diabetes is based on the background frequency of abnormal glucose metabolism in the population and on local circumstances.

According to NICE guidlines: Assess risk of gestational diabetes using risk factors in a healthy population. At the booking appointment, determine the following risk factors for gestational diabetes:

BMI above 30kg/m^2

Previous macrosomic baby weighing 4.5kg or above

Previous gestational diabetes

Family history of diabetes (first-degree relative with diabetes)

Minority ethnic family origin with a high prevalence of diabetes.

Offer women with any one of these risk factors testing for gestational diabetes.

(Do not use fasting plasma glucose, random blood glucose, HbA1c, glucose challenge test or urinalysis for glucose to assess risk of developing gestational diabetes)

(Be aware that glycosuria of 2+ or above on 1 occasion or of 1+ or above on 2 or more occasions detected by reagent strip testing during routine antenatal care may indicate undiagnosed gestational diabetes. If this is observed, consider further testing to exclude gestational diabetes)

(TESTING: 2-hour 75g oral glucose tolerance test (OGTT) to test for gestational diabetes in women with risk factors)

(Offer women who have had gestational diabetes in a previous pregnancy: early self-monitoring of blood glucose OR a 75g 2-hour OGTT as soon as possible after booking (whether in the first or second trimester), and a further 75g 2-hour OGTT at 24–28weeks if the results of the first OGTT are normal.)

(Offer women with any of the other risk factors for gestational diabetes a 75g 2-hour OGTT at 24–28weeks.)

Impact of overt (pre-gestational) diabetes on pregnancy:

Foetal effects:

a) Spontaneous abortions: HbA1c >7% or plasma glucose >120mg/dl associated with three fold increase in risk of spontaneous abortion.

b) Preterm delivery: 26% (6.8% in normal population) rate of preterm delivery in overt diabetic population.

c) Malformation: in type 1 DM incidence is double (5%). Half are cardiovascular anomalies (there is fourfold increase in cardiac anomalies as compared to non-cardiac anomalies). Incidence of various anomalies according to **Eidem** 2010 is:

Cardiovascular(52%), Musculoskeletal (12%), Urogenital (9%), CNS (4%), Gastrointestinal (2%), Chromosomal (3%), Other (10%), Multi-organ(8%). Although caudal regression is rare malformation it is frequently associated with maternal diabetes.

The frequency of major congenital malformation in new-born with pregestational diabetes according to HBA1c in first visit:

<6% HBA1c : 2.8%
6-6.9HBA1c% : 5%
7-7.9%HBA1c : 11.7%
8%HBA1c >= : 15.8%

Possible explanation is: Hyperglycaemia produces toxic radical and initiate programmed cell death. Also it is observed that hyperglycaemia oxidative stress inhibit migration of cardiac neural-crest cell in embryo of diabetic mice.

d) Altered foetal growth :

Diminished foetal growth: more typical of pre-gestational diabetes mellitus. Results from congenital malformation or from substrate deprivation due to advanced vascular disease.

Macrosomia: particularly in second half of gestation maternal hyperglycaemia prompts foetal hyperinsulinemia which cause macrosomia. Except brain most of part affected. There is deposition of fat on shoulder, trunk which may cause shoulder dystocia. Incidence of macrosomia rises with increase in maternal plasma glucose level more than 130mg/dl. Incidence of macrosomia in type 1, type 2 and gestational diabetes mellitus is 35%,28%,24%(in Noradic women) respectively.

e) Unexplained foetal demise:

Three times more in type 1 DM as compared to general obstetrical population. Stillbirths generally occur after 35 weeks before labour and babies are typically large for gestational age. The cause is unexplained (because common causes like obvious placental insufficiency, abruption, foetal growth restriction, or oligohydramnios are not identified). These unexplained stillbirth commonly (2/3rd of cases) associated with poor glycaemic control. According to Pedersen this may be due to hyperglycaemia mediated chronic aberrations in oxygen and foetal metabolic transport. This is supported by study conducted by Salvesen which show mean umbilical vein ph is less in diabetic pregnancy. Also there is 7 fold increase in unexplained stillbirth in pregnancy associated with both diabetes and PIH as compared to 3 fold increase in diabetes alone.

f) Hydramnios (AFI >24CM): women with elevated HbA1c and uncontrolled sugar level found to have more incidence of polyhydramnios in third trimester.
g) Neonatal effect: increased neonatal morbidity due to preterm birth and early induction to avoid unexplained stillbirth.
h) Respiratory distress syndrome: historically, new-borns of diabetic mothers were thought to be at increased risk for respiratory distress from delayed lung maturation. But recent study by **Bental** and colleague fails to demonstrate this concept. Gestational age is more important factor.
i) Hypoglycaemia: because of hyperplasia of beta islet cells induced by chronic maternal hyperglycaemia, new-born

of diabetic mother experience rapid drop in plasma glucose concentration. Low glycaemia defined by plasma glucose level below 45mg/dl. Prompt recognition and monitoring decrease incidence of hypoglycaemia.

j) Hypocalcaemia: it is defined as serum level less than 8 mg/dl in term neonates. Every third patient in uncontrolled diabetes mellitus developed hypocalcaemia as compared to controlled diabetes where incidence is 18%.

k) Hyperbilirubinemia and polycythaemia: polycythaemia is thought to be due to chronic hypoxia induced by hyperglycaemia. Hyperglycaemia in mother consumed more oxygen depriving foetus of oxygen. This hypoxia induces increase erythropoietin. Increase erythropoietin along with increase insulin cause polycythaemia. Polycythaemia cause increase bilirubin. 40 % of neonate show haematocrits of 65-70% volume.

l) Cardiomyopathy: primarily affect interventricular septum followed by right ventricle. In severe cases cardiomyopathy leads to obstructive cardiac failure. Structural changes precede cardiac failure. Most of affected new born asymptomatic at birth and hypertrophy resolved in months after birth because of relief from maternal hyperglycaemia. Conversely foetal cardiomyopathy may progress to adult cardiomyopathy.

m) Long term cognitive development:
Despite of rigorous antepartum management intelligence quotient (by 1 to 2 points) and memory is less in babies of mother with overt diabetes in pregnancy. Also incidence of autism is more.

n) Inheritance of diabetes: risk of developing type 1 if either parent affected is 3 or 4 %. If both parent have type 2 DM then incidence of inheritance is 40%. It is observed that breast feeding increase incidence of developing type 1 DM and decrease incidence of type 2 DM.

Maternal effects:

With possible exception of diabetic retinopathy the long term diabetes is not affected by pregnancy. Reported maternal mortality from type 1 DM is 0.5%. Death mostly result from diabetic ketoacidosis, hypoglycaemia, hypertension and infection.

Preeclampsia:

Incidence of preeclampsia is increased 3 to 4 times more often in women with overt diabetes. Diabetes with coexisting chronic hypertension has 12 times more incidence of developing preeclampsia. Especially risk factor for preeclampsia includes any vascular complications and pre-existing proteinuria, with or without chronic hypertension. Women in more advanced stage of White classification have more chances of developing preeclampsia. This increase in incidence was thought to be because of increase in oxidative stress. But supplementation with vitamin C and E do not decrease incidence. **Temple and co-worker** concluded in their study that incidence of preeclampsia is related to glycaemic control and HbA1c level.

Diabetic Nephropathy:

Clinically detectable nephropathy begins with micro albuminuria 30 to 300mg/24 hour, this may manifest as early as 5 years after diabetes onset. Macro albuminuria (more than 300mg/24 hour) develops in patient destined to have end stage renal disease. Hypertension develops in patient with macro albuminuria and renal failure ensues in typically in 5 to 10 years.

"Incidence of proteinuria is 30% in type 1DM and 4 to 20% in type 2 DM".

Well controlled blood sugar level can decrease incidence of diabetic nephropathy. There is 25% decrease in rate of nephropathy for each 10% decrease in haemoglobin HBA1c level. Approximately 5% of women with diabetes have renal involvement and 40 % of them develops preeclampsia. Although **How and colleagues** show no association of micro albuminuria to preeclampsia but they found increased risk of preeclampsia to 60% in cases of chronic hypertension with overt diabetic nephropathy. Mild renal impairment does not worsen with pregnancy but moderate and severe renal impairment worsen with pregnancy. Substantial proteinuria and hypertension are major predictive factor for progression to renal failure.

Diabetic retinopathy:

Retinal vasculopathy is highly specific complication of type 1 and type2 diabetes mellitus. First and most common sign is small aneurysm followed by blot haemorrhages that form when erythrocyte escape. These areas leak serous fluid which form hard exudates. This is known as *benign or non-proliferative or background retinopathy*. With increasing severity abnormal vessels of background retinopathy become occluded, leading to ischemia and infarction that appear as cotton wool exudates. This is called pre-proliferative retinopathy. Due to ischemia there is neovascularization on the retinal surface and out into vitreous cavity. Vision is obscured when there is haemorrhage. This is called proliferative retinopathy. About two third of women with type 1 DM have background retinopathy, proliferative retinopathy or macular oedema around 8 weeks of gestation and one fourth of them progress at least in one eye. While in type 2 DM only 14% have retinopathy and only 14% have progression. **Arun and Taylor** found that baseline retinopathy is independent risk factor for progression. Other risk factors include hypertension, higher level of insulin like growth factor and macular oedema early in pregnancy.

The National Institute for Health and Clinical Excellence (2008) established guidelines recommending that pregnant women with pre-existing diabetes should routinely be offered retinal assessment after the first prenatal visit. Currently, most agree that laser photocoagulation and good glycaemic control during pregnancy minimize the potential for deleterious effects of pregnancy. **Wang and co-workers** (1993) have observed that retinopathy worsened during the critical months of rigorous glucose control, but long term, deterioration of eye disease slowed.

Diabetic Neuropathy:

Peripheral symmetrical sensorimotor diabetic neuropathy is uncommon in pregnant women. But a form of this, known as diabetic gastropathy, is troublesome during pregnancy. It causes nausea and vomiting, nutritional problems, and difficulty with glucose control. Women with gastro paresis should be advised that this complication is associated with a high risk of morbidity and poor perinatal outcome **(Kitz miller**, 2008). Treatment with metoclopramide and H2-receptor antagonists is sometimes successful. Hyperemesis gravidarum worsens because of this.

Diabetic Ketoacidosis:

It is most often encountered in women with type 1 diabetes. Diabetic ketoacidosis (DKA) may develop with hyperemesis gravidarum, β-mimetic drugs given for tocolysis, infection, and corticosteroids given to induce foetal lung maturation. DKA results from an insulin deficiency combined with an excess in counter-regulatory hormones such as glucagon. This leads to gluconeogenesis and ketone body formation. The ketone body β-hydroxybutyrate is synthesized at a much greater rate than acetoacetate, which is preferentially detected by commonly used ketosis detection methodologies. Therefore, serum or plasma assays for β-hydroxybutyrate more accurately reflect true ketone body levels.

"The incidence of foetal loss can be as high as 20 percent with DKA". Pregnant women usually develop ketoacidosis at lower blood glucose thresholds than when nonpregnant. In a study from China, the mean glucose level for pregnant women with DKA was 293 mg/dl compared with 495 mg/dl for nonpregnant women (**Guo**, 2008). Chico and associates (2008) reported ketoacidosis in a pregnant woman whose plasma glucose was only 87 mg/dl.

Management of diabetes ketoacidosis

Management:

An important cornerstone of management is vigorous rehydration with crystalloid solutions of normal saline or ringer lactate.

Protocol Recommended by the American College of Obstetricians and Gynecologists (2012) for Management of Diabetic Ketoacidosis During Pregnancy

Laboratory assessment

Obtain arterial blood gases to document degree of acidosis present; measure glucose, ketones, and electrolyte levels at 1- to 2-hour intervals.

Insulin:

Low-dose, intravenous

Loading dose: 0.2–0.4 U/kg

Maintenance: 2–10 U/hr

Fluids:
Isotonic sodium chloride
Total replacement in first 12 hours of 4–6 L
1 L in first hour
500–1000 mL/hr for 2–4 hours
250 mL/hr until 80 percent replaced

Glucose: Begin 5-percent dextrose in normal saline when glucose plasma level reaches 250 mg/dL (14 mmol/L).

Potassium:
        If Initially normal or reduced, an infusion rate up to 15–20 mEq/hr may be required; if elevated, wait until levels decrease into the normal range, then add to intravenous solution in a concentration of 20–30 mEq/L

Bicarbonate:
        Add one ampule (44 mEq) to 1 L of 0.45 normal saline if pH is < 7.1

Infections:

Stamler and Coworkers (1990) reported that almost 80 % of women with type 1 diabetes develop at least one infection during pregnancy compared with only 25 % in those without diabetes. Common infections include Candida vulvovaginitis, urinary and respiratory tract infections, and puerperal pelvic sepsis. Positive urine cultures in a fourth of diabetic women compared with 10 % of nondiabetic pregnant women. 5 percent of women with diabetes developed pyelonephritis compared with 1.3% of the nondiabetic population. **Takoudes and colleagues** (2004) found that pregestational diabetes is associated with a two- to threefold increase in wound complications after caesarean delivery.

Management of Diabetes in Pregnancy

Preconception Care:

The ADA has defined optimal pre-conception glucose control using insulin to include self-monitored pre-prandial glucose levels of 70 to 100 mg/dl, peak postprandial values of 100 to 129 mg/dl, and   mean daily glucose concentrations < 110 mg/dl (**Kitz miller**, 2008). Glycosylated haemoglobin measurement, which reflects an average of circulating glucose for the past 4 to 8 weeks, is useful to assess early metabolic control. The ADA (2012) defines optimal values to be < 7 percent. A substantial fourfold increased risk for malformations at levels > 10 percent is found. If indicated, evaluation and treatment for diabetic complications such as retinopathy or nephropathy should also be instituted before pregnancy. Folate 400 µg/day orally is given in peri-conceptional period and during early pregnancy to decrease the risk of neural-tube defects.

First Trimester:

Careful monitoring of glucose control is essential. So hospitalize overtly diabetic women during early pregnancy to initiate an individualized glucose control program and offer education. It also provides an opportunity to assess the extent of diabetic vascular complications and precisely establish gestational age.

Insulin Treatment:

The overtly diabetic pregnant woman is best treated with insulin. Although oral hypoglycaemic agents have been used successfully for gestational diabetes, these agents are not currently recommended for overt diabetes except for limited and individualized use (American College of Obstetricians and Gynecologists, 2012). Maternal glycaemic control can usually be achieved with multiple daily insulin injections and adjustment of dietary intake. The action profiles of commonly used short- and long-term insulin are shown in table:

Insulin type	Onset	Peak (hours)	Duration (hours)
Short acting (SC)			
Lispro	<15 Min	0.5-1.5	3-4
Glulisine	<15 Min	0.5-1.5	3-4
Aspart	<15 Min	0.5-1.5	3-4
Regular	30-60 min	2-3	4-6
Long acting			
Detemir	1-4 hour	Minimal	Up to 24
Glargine	1-4 hour	Minimal	Up to 24
NPH	1-4 hour	6-10	10-16

Insulin pump can also be used in pregnancy. In a met-analysis of six small randomized trials comparing insulin pumps to multiple daily injections of insulin, there were no significant differences in LGA birth weight, maternal hypoglycaemia, or retinopathy progression (Mukhopadhyay, 2007). Notably, more women using insulin pumps developed ketoacidosis. Women who use an insulin pump must be highly motivated and compliant to minimize the risk of nocturnal hypoglycaemia **(Gabbe**, 2003).

Monitoring:

Self-monitoring of capillary glucose levels using a glucometer is recommended. Glucose goals recommended during pregnancy are:

Specimen	Mg/dl
Fasting	5.3mmol/litre (96mg/dl)
1 hour postprandial	7.8mmol/litre (140mg/dl)
2 hour postprandial	6.4mmol/litre (116mg/dl)

Monitoring blood glucose:

1. Advise pregnant women with type1 diabetes to test their fasting, pre-meal, 1-hour post-meal and bedtime blood glucose levels daily during pregnancy.

2. Advise pregnant women with type2 diabetes or gestational diabetes who are on a multiple daily insulin injection regimen to

test their fasting, pre-meal, 1-hour post-meal and bedtime blood glucose levels daily during pregnancy.

3. Advise pregnant women with type2 diabetes or gestational diabetes to test their fasting and 1-hour post-meal blood glucose levels daily during pregnancy if they are:

-on diet and exercise therapy

-taking oral therapy (with or without diet and exercise therapy) or single-dose intermediate-acting or long-acting insulin

Diet:

The mix of carbohydrate, protein, and fat is adjusted to meet the metabolic goals and individual patient preferences, but a 175-g minimum of carbohydrate per day should be provided. Carbohydrate should be distributed throughout the day in three small- to moderate-sized meals and two to four snacks **(Bantle**, 2008). Weight loss is not recommended, but modest caloric restriction may be appropriate for overweight or obese women. An ideal dietary composition is 55 percent carbohydrate, 20 percent protein, and 25 percent fat, of which < 10 percent is saturated fat.

Hypoglycaemia:

Chen and co-workers (2007) identified hypoglycaemic events—blood glucose < 40 mg/dl—in 37 of 60 women with type 1 - diabetes. **Rosenn and colleagues** (1994) noted that maternal hypoglycaemia had a peak incidence between 10 and 15 weeks' gestation. Caution is recommended when attempting euglycaemia in women with recurrent episodes of hypoglycaemia.

Second Trimester:

Maternal serum alpha-fetoprotein determination at 16 to 20 weeks' gestation and targeted sonographic examination at 18 to 20 weeks to detect neural-tube defects and other anomalies. Maternal alpha-fetoprotein levels may be lower in diabetic pregnancies, and interpretation is altered accordingly. As the incidence of congenital cardiac anomalies is five times greater in mothers with diabetes, foetal echocardiography is an important part of second trimester sonographic evaluation.

Euglycaemia with self-monitoring continues to be the goal in management. After the first-trimester instability, a stable period ensues. This is followed by an increased insulin requirement. **Roeder and co-worker**s (2012) identified a threefold increase in total daily insulin after the first trimester in women using an insulin pump. This is due to the increased peripheral resistance to insulin.

Third Trimester and Delivery:

From early third trimester women should attend OPD every 2 weeks. During these visits, glycaemic control is evaluated and insulin adjusted. They are routinely instructed to perform foetal kick counts beginning early in the third trimester. NICE guidelines suggest initiation of antenatal foetal surveillance at 32 to 34 weeks' gestation. It includes foetal movement counting, periodic foetal heart rate monitoring, intermittent biophysical profile evaluation, and contraction stress testing. At 34 weeks, admission is offered to all insulin-treated women. While in the hospital, they continue daily foetal movement counts and undergo foetal heart rate monitoring three times a week. Delivery is planned for 38 weeks.

Labour induction may be attempted when the foetus is not excessively large and the cervix is considered favourable. Cesarean delivery at or near term has frequently been used to avoid traumatic birth of a large infant in a woman with diabetes. In a nested case-control study of 209 women with type 1 diabetes, **Leper and colleagues** (2010) reported a 70-percent cesarean delivery rate overall. Two thirds of these were delivered without labour. Both maternal body mass index (BMI) > 25 kg/m2 and low Bishop Score were independently associated with cesarean delivery for those in labour. In another study, a glycohemoglobin level > 6.4 percent at delivery was independently associated with urgent cesarean delivery. This suggests that tighter glycaemic control during the third trimester might reduce late foetal compromise and cesarean delivery for foetal indications **(Miailhe,** 2013). Reducing or withholding the dose of long-acting insulin given on the day of delivery is recommended. Regular insulin should be used to meet most or all of the insulin needs of the mother during this time, because insulin requirements typically drop markedly after delivery. Continuous insulin infusion by calibrated intravenous pump is most satisfactory. Throughout labour and after delivery, the woman should be adequately hydrated intravenously and given glucose in sufficient amounts to maintain normoglycemia. Capillary or plasma glucose levels should be checked frequently, especially during active labour, and regular insulin should be administered accordingly.

Insulin Management during Labour and Delivery :

• Usual dose of intermediate-acting insulin is given at bedtime.
• Morning dose of insulin is withheld.
• Intravenous infusion of normal saline is begun.
• Once active labour begins or glucose levels decrease to < 70 mg/dl, the infusion is changed from saline to 5-percent dextrose and delivered at a rate of 100–150 mL/hr. (2.5 mg/kg/min) to achieve a glucose level of approximately 100 mg/dl.
• Glucose levels are checked hourly using a bedside meter allowing for adjustment in the insulin or glucose infusion rate.
• Regular (short-acting) insulin is administered by intravenous infusion at a rate of 1.25 U/hr if glucose levels exceed 100 mg/dl.

Puerperium:

Often, women may require virtually no insulin for the first 24 hours or so postpartum. Infection must be promptly detected and treated. Counselling in the Puerperium should include a discussion of birth control.

Refer women with pre-existing diabetes back to their routine diabetes care arrangements.

NICE protocol for weekly management of pregnancy with diabetes mellitus:

Appointment	Care for women with diabetes during pregnancy
Booking appointment (joint diabetes and antenatal care) – ideally by 10weeks	Discuss information, education and advice about how diabetes will affect the pregnancy, birth and early parenting (such as breastfeeding and initial care of the baby). If the woman has been attending for preconception care and advice, continue to provide information, education and advice in relation to achieving optimal blood

	glucose control (including dietary advice). If the woman has not attended for preconception care and advice, give information, education and advice for the first time, take a clinical history to establish the extent of diabetes-related complications (including neuropathy and vascular disease), and review medicines for diabetes and its complications. Offer retinal assessment for women with pre-existing diabetes unless the woman has been assessed in the last 3months. Offer renal assessment for women with pre-existing diabetes if this has not been performed in the last 3months. Arrange contact with the joint diabetes and antenatal clinic every 1–2weeks throughout pregnancy for all women with diabetes. Measure HbA1c levels for women with pre-existing diabetes to determine the level of risk for the pregnancy. Offer self-monitoring of blood glucose or a 75g 2-hour OGTT as soon as possible for women with a history of gestational diabetes who book in the first trimester. Confirm viability of pregnancy and gestational age at 7–9weeks.
16weeks	Offer retinal assessment at 16–20weeks to women with pre-existing diabetes if diabetic retinopathy was present at their first antenatal clinic visit. Offer self-monitoring of blood glucose or a 75g 2-hour OGTT as soon as possible for women with a history of gestational diabetes who book in the second trimester.
20weeks	Offer an ultrasound scan for detecting foetal structural abnormalities, including examination of the foetal heart (4chambers, outflow tracts and 3 vessels).
28weeks	Offer ultrasound monitoring of foetal growth and amniotic fluid volume. Offer retinal assessment to all women with pre-existing diabetes. Women diagnosed with

	gestational diabetes as a result of routine antenatal testing at 24–28weeks enter the care pathway.
32weeks	Offer ultrasound monitoring of foetal growth and amniotic fluid volume. Offer nulliparous women all routine investigations normally scheduled for 31weeks in routine antenatal care.
34weeks	No additional or different care for women with diabetes.
36weeks	Offer ultrasound monitoring of foetal growth and amniotic fluid volume. Provide information and advice about: timing, mode and management of birth analgesia and anaesthesia changes to blood glucose-lowering therapy during and after birth care of the baby after birth initiation of breastfeeding and the effect of breastfeeding on blood glucose control contraception and follow-up.
37+0 weeks to 38+6 weeks	Offer induction of labour, or caesarean section if indicated, to women with type1 or type2 diabetes; otherwise await spontaneous labour.
38weeks	Offer tests of foetal wellbeing.
39weeks	Offer tests of foetal wellbeing. Advise women with uncomplicated gestational diabetes to give birth no later than 40+6 weeks.

* Women with diabetes should also receive routine care according to the schedule of appointments in the NICE guideline on antenatal care, including appointments at 25weeks (for nulliparous women) and 34weeks, but with the exception of the appointment for nulliparous women at 31weeks. OGTT = oral glucose tolerance test.

GES

Gestational Diabetes Mellitus

Gestational diabetes is defined as carbohydrate intolerance of variable severity with onset or first recognition during pregnancy (American College of Obstetricians and Gynecologists, 2013). More than half of women with gestational diabetes ultimately develop overt diabetes in the ensuing 20 years.

Screening:

According to NICE guidlines: Assess risk of gestational diabetes using risk factors in a healthy population. At the booking appointment, determine the following risk factors for gestational diabetes:

BMI above 30kg/m^2

Previous macrosomic baby weighing 4.5kg or above

Previous gestational diabetes

Family history of diabetes (first-degree relative with diabetes)

Minority ethnic family origin with a high prevalence of diabetes.

Offer women with any one of these risk factors testing for gestational diabetes.

(Do not use fasting plasma glucose, random blood glucose, HbA1c, glucose challenge test or urinalysis for glucose to assess risk of developing gestational diabetes)

(Be aware that glycosuria of 2+ or above on 1 occasion or of 1+ or above on 2 or more occasions detected by reagent strip testing during routine antenatal care may indicate undiagnosed gestational diabetes. If this is observed, consider further testing to exclude gestational diabetes)

(TESTING: 2-hour 75g oral glucose tolerance test (OGTT) to test for gestational diabetes in women with risk factors)

(Offer women who have had gestational diabetes in a previous pregnancy: early self-monitoring of blood glucose OR a 75g 2-hour OGTT as soon as possible after booking (whether in the first or second trimester), and a further 75g 2-hour OGTT at 24–28weeks if the results of the first OGTT are normal.)

(Offer women with any of the other risk factors for gestational diabetes a 75g 2-hour OGTT at 24–28weeks.)

NICE Guideline for diagnosis:

Diagnose gestational diabetes if the woman has either:

-A fasting plasma glucose level of 5.6mmol/litre (100mg/dl) or above

-A 2-hour plasma glucose level of 7.8mmol/litre (140mg/dl) or above

Maternal and foetal effects of gestational diabetes mellitus:

Adverse consequences of gestational diabetes differ from those of pre-gestational diabetes. Unlike in women with overt diabetes, rates of **foetal anomalies do not appear** to be substantially increased.

The **stillbirth rate is not increase** as compared to non-diabetic population in well controlled sugar level. It is observed that women with elevated fasting glucose levels have increased rates of unexplained stillbirths similar to women with overt diabetes. The ADA (2003) concluded that fasting hyperglycaemia > 105 mg/dl may be associated with an increased risk of foetal death during the final 4 to 8 weeks.

Similar to women with overt diabetes, adverse maternal effects associated with gestational diabetes include an **increased frequency of hypertension and caesarean** delivery.

Foetal Macrosomia: Landon and colleagues (2011) identified shoulder dystocia in approximately 4 percent of women with mild gestational diabetes compared with < 1 percent of women with a 50-g glucose screen result < 120 mg/dl. In a prospective study of foetal adipose measurements, however, **Buhling and coworkers** (2012) demonstrated no differences between measurements in 630 offspring of women with gestational diabetes and 142 without diabetes. The authors attributed this negative finding to successful treatment of gestational diabetes. There is extensive evidence that insulin-like growth factors also play a role foetal-growth regulation. These proinsulin-like polypeptides are produced by virtually all foetal organs and are potent stimulators of cell differentiation and division. **Luo and coworkers** (2012) reported that insulin-like growth factor-I strongly correlated with birth weight. The HAPO study investigators also reported dramatic increases of cord-serum C-peptide levels with increasing maternal glucose levels following a 75-g OGTT. C-peptide levels > 90th percentile were found in almost a third of new-borns in the highest glucose categories. Other factors implicated in macrosomia include epidermal growth factor, fibroblast growth factor, platelet-derived growth factor, leptin and adiponectin (**Grissa,** 2011; **Loukovaara, 2004; Mazaki-Tovi, 2005**).

Neonatal Hypoglycaemia:

New-borns described by the HAPO study (2008) had an incidence of clinical neonatal hypoglycaemia that increased with increasing maternal OGTT values. The frequency varied from 1 to 2 percent, but it was as high as 4.6 percent in women with fasting glucose levels ≥ 100 mg/dl. Likewise, cord-blood insulin levels are related to maternal glucose control (**Leipold,** 2004).

Maternal Obesity: In women with gestational diabetes, maternal BMI is an independent and more substantial risk factor for foetal macrosomia than is glucose intolerance (Ehrenberg, 2004; Mission, 2013). In their metaanalysis, **Torloni and coworkers** (2009) estimated that the gestational diabetes prevalence increases by approximately 1 percent for every 1 kg/m2 increase in BMI. Weight distribution also seems to play a role because the risk of gestational diabetes is increased with truncal obesity. Suresh and colleagues (2012) verified that increased maternal abdominal subcutaneous fat thickness as measured by sonography at 18 to 22 weeks' gestation correlated with BMI and was a better predictor of gestational diabetes.

Management of gestational diabetes mellitus

Pharmacological methods are usually recommended if diet modification does not consistently maintain the fasting plasma glucose levels < 95 mg/dl or the 2-hour postprandial plasma glucose < 120 mg/dl (American College of Obstetricians and Gynecologists, 2013). Whether pharmacological treatment should be used in women with lesser degrees of fasting hyperglycaemia— 105 mg/dl or less before dietary intervention—is unclear. In a systematic review, **Hartling and colleagues** (2013) concluded that treating gestational diabetes resulted in a significantly lower incidence of preeclampsia, shoulder dystocia, and macrosomia. they were unable to demonstrate an effect on neonatal hypoglycaemia or future metabolic outcomes in the offspring.

Patient Education: The importance of educating women with GDM (and their partners) about the condition and its management cannot be overemphasized. The compliance with the treatment plan depends on the patient's understanding of:

- The implications of GDM for her baby and herself

-The dietary and exercise recommendations

-Self monitoring of blood glucose

- Self administration of insulin and adjustment of insulin doses

- Identification and treatment of hypoglycaemia (patient and family members)

- Incorporate safe physical activity

-Development of techniques to reduce stress and cope with the denial. Care should be taken to minimise the anxiety of the women.

Preconception care:

-Advice women with diabetes who are planning to become pregnant to aim to keep their HbA1c level below 48mmol/l (6.5%), if this is achievable without causing problematic hypoglycaemia.

-Strongly advise women with diabetes whose HbA1c level is above 86mmol/l (10%) not to get pregnant because of the associated risks.

- Offer women with diabetes a renal assessment, including a measure of low-level albuminuria (micro albuminuria), before discontinuing contraception. If serum creatinine is abnormal (120mmol/litre or more), the urinary albumin:creatinine ratio is greater than 30mg/mmol or the estimated glomerular filtration rate (eGFR) is less than 45ml/minute/1.73m^2, referral to a nephrologist should be considered before discontinuing contraception.

- Carry out retinal assessment by digital imaging with mydriasis using tropicamide, in line with the UK National Screening Committee's recommendations for annual mydriatic 2-field digital photographic screening as part of a systematic screening programme.

Diabetic Diet: Nutritional instructions generally include a carbohydrate-controlled diet sufficient to maintain normoglycemia and avoid ketosis. On average, this includes a daily caloric intake of 30 to 35 kcal/kg. Carbohydrate intake be limited to 40 percent of total calories. The remaining calories are apportioned to give 20 percent as protein and 40 percent as fat. Although the most appropriate diet for women with gestational diabetes has not been established, the ADA (2003) has suggested that obese women with a BMI > 30 kg/m2 may benefit from a 30percent caloric restriction, which approximates 25 kcal/kg/d. This should be monitored with weekly assessment for ketonuria, which has been linked with impaired psychomotor development in offspring.

Foods with a low glycaemic index should replace those with a high glycaemic index.

EXERCISE: Dempsey and co-workers (2004) found that physical activity during pregnancy reduced the risk of gestational diabetes. **Brankston and associates** (2004) reported that resistance exercise diminished the need for insulin therapy in overweight women with gestational diabetes. Conversely, **Stafne and colleagues** (2012), in a randomized controlled trial in 855 women, observed that a 1-week exercise program during the second half of pregnancy did not prevent gestational diabetes or improve insulin resistance. Advise women with gestational diabetes to take regular exercise (such as walking for 30minutes after a meal) to improve blood glucose control. Importantly, the average BMI at enrolment was 24.8 ± 3.2.

Medical Nutrition Therapy (MNT)

Offer a trial of changes in diet and exercise to women with gestational diabetes **who have a fasting plasma glucose level below 7mmol/litre (126mg/dl)** at diagnosis. Offer metformin to women with gestational diabetes if blood glucose targets are not met using changes in diet and exercise within 1–2weeks. Offer addition of insulin to the treatments of changes in diet, exercise and metformin for women with gestational diabetes if blood glucose targets are not met.

a) General Principles: All women with GDM should receive nutritional counselling. The meal pattern should provide adequate calories and nutrients to meet the needs of pregnancy. The expected weight gain during pregnancy is 300 to 400 gm/week and total weight gain is 10 to 12 kg by term. Hence the meal plan aims to provide sufficient calories to sustain adequate nutrition for the mother and foetus and to avoid excess weight gain and post prandial hyperglycaemia. Calorie requirement depends on age, activity, pre pregnancy weight and stage of pregnancy. Approximately 30 to 40 Kcal/kg ideal body weight or an increment of 300 kcal/day above the basal requirement is needed. Pregnancy is not the ideal time for obesity correction. Underweight subjects or those not gaining weight as expected, particularly in the third trimester, require admission to ensure adequate nutrition to prevent low birth weight infants.

b) Calorie Counting: As a part of the medical nutrition therapy, pregnant diabetic woman are advised to wisely distribute their calorie consumption especially the breakfast. This implies splitting the usual breakfast into two equal halves and consuming the portions with a two hour gap in between. By this the undue peak in plasma glucose levels after ingestion of the total quantity of breakfast at one time is avoided. For example if 4 idles / chapatti / slices of bread (applies to all type of breakfast menu) is taken for breakfast at 8 am and two hours plasma glucose at 10 am is 140mg:

the same quantity divided into two equal portions i.e., one portion at 8 am and remaining after 10 am, the two hours post prandial plasma glucose at 10.00 am falls by 20 – 30 mg.

This advice has scientific basis as the peaking of plasma glucose is high with breakfast (due to Dawn phenomenon) than with lunch and dinner. Further in a normal person, insulin secretion is also high with breakfast than with lunch or dinner. GDM mothers have deficiency in first phase insulin secretion and to match this insulin deficiency the challenge of quantity of food at one time should also be less

Glucose Monitoring: Women using daily blood-glucose self-monitoring had significantly fewer macrosomic infants and gained less weight after diagnosis than women evaluated during clinic visits only. Postprandial surveillance was shown to be superior in that blood-glucose control was significantly improved and was associated with fewer cases of neonatal hypoglycaemia—3 versus 21%; less macrosomia—12 versus 42%; and fewer caesarean deliveries for dystocia—24 versus 39 percent. The

Monitoring blood glucose:

1. Advise pregnant women with type1 diabetes to test their fasting, pre-meal, 1-hour post-meal and bedtime blood glucose levels daily during pregnancy.

2. Advise pregnant women with type2 diabetes or gestational diabetes who are on a multiple daily insulin injection regimen to test their fasting, pre-meal, 1-hour post-meal and bedtime blood glucose levels daily during pregnancy.

3. Advise pregnant women with type2 diabetes or gestational diabetes to test their fasting and 1-hour post-meal blood glucose levels daily during pregnancy if they are:

-on diet and exercise therapy

-taking oral therapy (with or without diet and exercise therapy) or single-dose intermediate-acting or long-acting insulin

Insulin Treatment: Historically, insulin has been considered standard therapy in women with gestational diabetes when target glucose levels cannot be consistently achieved through nutrition and exercise. It does not cross the placenta, and tight glycaemic control can typically be achieved.

Offer immediate treatment with insulin, with or without metformin, as well as changes in diet and exercise, to women with gestational diabetes who have a fasting plasma glucose level of 7.0mmol/litre(126mg/dl) or above at diagnosis.

Consider immediate treatment with insulin, with or without metformin, as well as changes in diet and exercise, for women with gestational diabetes who have a fasting plasma glucose level of between 6.0 and 6.9mmol/litre(108 to 124mg/dl) if there are complications such as macrosomia or hydramnios.

If insulin is initiated, the starting dose is typically 0.7–1.0 units/kg/day given in divided doses (American College of Obstetricians and Gynecologists, 2013). A combination of intermediate-acting and short-acting insulin may be used, and dose adjustments are based on glucose levels at particular times of the day. , insulin analogues such as insulin aspart and insulin lispro have a more rapid onset of action than regular insulin and theoretically could be helpful in postprandial glucose management.

The initial dose of NPH insulin could be as low as 4 units and the dose of insulin can be adjusted on follow up. A few GDM patients may require combination of short acting insulin and intermediate acting insulin in the morning and evening.

1) If a patient has elevated pre-lunch blood sugar, regular insulin is usually necessary in the morning to handle the post breakfast hyperglycaemia, as there is a lag period before the intermediate-acting insulin begins to work. The above regimen of regular and intermediate-acting insulin in the morning controls hyperglycaemia in most cases.
2) If the post dinner blood sugar is high, a small dose of regular insulin is necessary before dinner in addition to the regular and intermediate acting insulin given in the morning.
3) Combination of regular and intermediate acting insulin before dinner may be necessary if fasting blood sugar is high. This combination of short and intermediate acting

insulin in the morning and as well as in the evening is known as mixed and split dose of insulin regimen. In this regimen two-third of the total daily dose of insulin is given in the morning and one third in the evening. For each combination one-third dose should be regular insulin and two-third intermediate acting insulin. With this regimen if the patient continues to have fasting hyperglycaemia, the intermediate acting insulin has to be given at bedtime instead of before dinner. Insulin dose is individualized.

Target Blood Glucose Levels:

Advise pregnant women with any form of diabetes to maintain their capillary plasma glucose below the following target levels, if these are achievable without causing problematic hypoglycaemia:

Fasting: 5.3mmol/litre (96mg/dl)

And

1hour after meals: 7.8mmol/litre (140mg/dl)

2hours after meals: 6.4mmol/litre (116mg/dl)

Advise pregnant women with diabetes who are on insulin or glibenclamide to maintain their capillary plasma glucose level above 4mmol/litre (72mg/dl). (MPG should not be < 86 mg/dl as this may cause small for gestational age infants).

Test urgently for ketonaemia if a pregnant woman with any form of diabetes presents with hyperglycaemia or is unwell, to exclude diabetic ketoacidosis

Species of Insulin:

It is ideal to use human insulin (least immunogenic). Though insulin does not cross the placenta, the insulin antibodies due to animal source insulin can cross the placenta, and stress the foetal beta cell, increase insulin production and induce macrosomia. Rapid acting insulin analogues, (**Novorapid/Humalog**) have been found to be safe and effective in achieving the targeted post prandial glucose value during pregnancy. Lispro the first analogue to get category B approval by US FDA and aspart has also been used in pregnancy.

Oral Hypoglycaemic Agents: The American College of Obstetricians and Gynecologists (2013) acknowledges that both glyburide and metformin are appropriate, as is insulin, for first-line glycaemic control in women with gestational diabetes. Because long-term outcomes have not been studied, the committee recommends appropriate counselling when hypoglycaemic agents are used. In their systematic review and metaanalysis of oral hypoglycaemic agents for gestational diabetes, **Nicholson and co-workers** (2009) found no evidence of increased adverse maternal or neonatal outcomes with glyburide or metformin compared with insulin. **Moore and associates** (2010) randomly assigned 149 women with gestational diabetes who did not achieve glycaemic control on diet therapy to either glyburide or metformin treatment. More than a third of women in the metformin group required supplemental insulin compared with 16 percent of those treated with glyburide.

NICE guidelines: Consider Glibenclamide for women with gestational diabetes:

-in whom blood glucose targets are not achieved with metformin but who decline insulin therapy.

-who cannot tolerate metformin.

Other parameters to be monitored during prgegnancy:

The blood pressure has to be monitored during every visit. Examination of the fundus and estimation of micro albuminuria, every trimester is recommended.

If renal assessment has not been undertaken in the preceding 3months in women with pre-existing diabetes, arrange it at the first contact in pregnancy. If the serum creatinine is abnormal (120micromol/litre or more), the urinary albumin:creatinine ratio is greater than 30mg/mmol or total protein excretion exceeds 2g/day, referral to a nephrologist should be considered (eGFR should not be used during pregnancy). Thrombo-prophylaxis should be considered for women with proteinuria above 5g/day (macro albuminuria).

Offer pregnant women with pre-existing diabetes retinal assessment by digital imaging with mydriasis using tropicamide following their first antenatal clinic appointment (unless they have had a retinal assessment in the last 3months), and again at 28weeks. If any diabetic retinopathy is present at booking, perform an additional retinal assessment at 16–20week. Diabetic retinopathy should not be considered a contraindication to vaginal birth.

Offer pregnant women with type1 diabetes blood ketone testing strips and a meter, and advise them to test for ketonaemia and to seek urgent medical advice if they become hyperglycaemic or unwell.

Advise pregnant women with type2 diabetes or gestational diabetes to seek urgent medical advice if they become hyperglycaemic or unwell.

Test urgently for ketonaemia if a pregnant woman with any form of diabetes presents with hyperglycaemia or is unwell, to exclude diabetic ketoacidosis.

Ultrasound: An ultrasound scan has to be performed around 18 – 20 weeks of gestation focusing on structures namely the spine, skull, kidney and heart. Foetal echocardiography has to be done around 20 – 24 weeks which allows to view all the four chambers of the heart. From 26th week onwards, foetal growth and liquor volume has to be monitored every 2-3 weeks. Foetal abdominal circumference provides baseline for further serial measurements which gives growth acceleration or restriction. Foetal movements are monitored from 20 weeks onwards. Screening for chromosomal anomalies is necessary in pre GDM. Screening should be done for Down's syndrome, α-feto protein for neural defects and human chorionic gonadotropin to identify any chromosomal abnormalities (16 – 20 weeks of gestation).

Obstetrical Management:

In general, for women with gestational diabetes who do not require insulin, early delivery or other interventions are seldom required. There is no consensus regarding the value or timing of antepartum foetal testing. It is typically reserved for women with pregestational diabetes because of the increased stillbirth risk. But it is always better for women with diabetes in pregnancy to start antepartum foetal monitoring early in third trimester. Insulin-treated women should be offered inpatient admission after 34 weeks' gestation, and foetal heart rate monitoring should be performed three times each week.

Women with gestational diabetes and adequate glycaemic control are managed expectantly. Elective labour induction to prevent shoulder dystocia compared with spontaneous labour remains controversial. It is observed that elective induction at 38 weeks results in lower incidence of macrosomia and there are no differences in rates of caesarean delivery or shoulder dystocia or in neonatal outcomes as compared to waiting for spontaneous labour. Most still advocate delivery at 38 weeks as perinatal mortality and morbidity appear to increase after this time. Induction at 38 weeks gestation may be slow or unsuccessful due to unfavourable conditions of the cervix but this has to be balanced against the poorly defined and predictable risk of late intra uterine death, if pregnancy is allowed to continue more than 38 weeks. Foetal health may deteriorate suddenly, hence obstetric management should not be rigid and each case needs individual care and attention. Having a neonatologist support at the time of delivery is advisable The American College of Obstetricians and Gynecologists (2013) has suggested that caesarean delivery should be considered in women with gestational diabetes whose foetuses have a sonographically estimated weight ≥ 4500 g.

Preterm labour in women with gestational diabetes mellitus

Diabetes should not be considered a contraindication to antenatal steroids for foetal lung maturation or to tocolysis.

In women with insulin-treated diabetes who are receiving steroids for foetal lung maturation, give additional insulin according to an agreed protocol and monitor them closely.

Do not use beta-mimetic medicines for tocolysis in women with diabetes.

*NICE guidelines: Advise pregnant women with **type1 or type2 diabetes and no other complications** to have an elective birth by induction of labour, or by elective caesarean section if indicated, between **37+0 weeks and 38+6** weeks of pregnancy. Advise women with **gestational diabetes** to give birth no later than **40+6 weeks**, and offer elective birth (by induction of labour, or by caesarean section if indicated) to women who have not given birth by this time.*

Intra Partum Management:

If labour is to be induced in GDM, the usual evening insulin dose should be taken the night before, but no subcutaneous insulin is given the following morning when induction begins.

Once labour begins, insulin is not necessary.

In a gestational diabetic the requirement of insulin is likely to fall precipitously and no insulin may be required immediately after expulsion of placenta.

Monitor capillary plasma glucose every hour during labour and birth in women with diabetes, and ensure that it is maintained between 4 mmol/litre (72mg/dl) to 7mmol/litre (126mg/dl).

Intravenous dextrose and insulin infusion should be considered for women with type1 diabetes from the onset of established labour.

Use intravenous dextrose and insulin infusion during labour and birth for women with diabetes whose capillary plasma glucose is not maintained between 4(72mg/dl) to 7(126mg/dl) mmol/litre.

Anaesthesia:

Offer women with diabetes and comorbidities such as obesity or autonomic neuropathy an anaesthetic assessment in the third trimester of pregnancy.

If general anaesthesia is used for the birth in women with diabetes, monitor blood glucose every 30minutes from induction of general anaesthesia until after the baby is born and the woman is fully conscious.

Delivery:

A paediatrician experienced in resuscitation of the newborn should be present whether delivery is vaginal or by caesarean section.

As soon as the infant is born, the following actions are mandatory:

-Early clamping of the cord, i.e. within 20 seconds of delivery, to avoid erythrocytosis.

-Evaluate vital signs; Apgar scores at 1 and 5 minutes;

-Clear oropharynx and nose of mucus; later empty the stomach - be aware that stimulation of the pharynx with the catheter may lead to reflex bradycardia and apnoea;

-Avoid heat loss, keep neonate warm, and transfer to incubator pre-warmed to 34^0C;

-Perform a preliminary physical examination to detect major congenital malformations;

-Monitor heart and respiratory rates, colour, and motor behaviour for at least the first 24 hours after birth;

-Women with diabetes should feed their babies as soon as possible after birth (within 30minutes) and then at frequent intervals (every 2–3hours) until feeding maintains pre-feed capillary plasma glucose levels at a minimum of 2.0mmol/litre(36mg/dl). Aim at full caloric intake (125 kcal/kg/24 hours) at 5 days, divided into six to eight feeds a day.

-Carry out blood glucose testing routinely in babies of women with diabetes at 2–4hours after birth. Carry out blood tests for polycythaemia, hyperbilirubinaemia, hypocalcaemia and hypomagnesaemia for babies with clinical signs. Perform an echocardiogram for babies of women with diabetes if they show clinical signs associated with congenital heart disease or cardiomyopathy, including heart murmur. The timing of the examination will depend on the clinical circumstances.

-If capillary plasma glucose values are below 2.0mmol/litre on 2consecutive readings despite maximal support for feeding, if there are abnormal clinical signs or if the baby will not feed orally effectively, use additional measures such as tube feeding or intravenous dextrose. Only implement additional measures if one or more of these criteria are met.

-Promote early infant-parent relationship (bonding).

-The neonate is usually best cared for, in a specialized neonatal unit. Interference with the infant should be minimal. The neonate should be observed closely after delivery for respiratory distress.

-Amperometric blood glucose meters are acceptable for use in neonates, provided that suitable quality-control procedures and operator training are in place. The cut-off of 44mg% (2.6 mmol/l) is now currently used as the working definition for hypoglycaemia. This "Operational threshold" is not a diagnosis of a disease but an indication for action. If the baby is obviously macrosomic, calcium and magnesium levels should be checked on day 2. Breastfeeding, as always, should be encouraged in women with GDM.

Postpartum Evaluation:

GDM may be viewed as:

1. An unidentified pre-existing disease, or

2. The unmasking of a compensated metabolic abnormality by the added stress of pregnancy, or

3. A direct consequence of the altered maternal metabolism stemming from the changing hormonal milieu.

Gestational diabetic women require follow up. Glucose tolerance test with 75g oral glucose is performed after 6 weeks of delivery and if necessary repeated after 6 months and every year to determine whether the glucose tolerance has returned to normal or progressed. A small proportion of gestational diabetic women may continue to have glucose intolerance.

Recommendations for postpartum evaluation are based on the 50-percent likelihood of women with gestational diabetes developing overt diabetes within 20 years (O'Sullivan, 1982).

Fifth International Workshop-Conference: Metabolic Assessments Recommended after Pregnancy with Gestational Diabetes		
Post-delivery (1-3days)	Fasting or random blood sugar	Detect persistence or overt diabetes
Early post-partum(6-12weeks)	75 gram 2 hr. OGTT	Post-partum classification of glucose metabolism
1-yr postpartum	75 gram 2 hr. OGTT	Assess glucose metabolism
Annually	Fasting blood sugar	Assess glucose metabolism
Tri-annually	75 gram 2 hr. OGTT	Assess glucose metabolism
Prepregnancy	75 gram 2 hr. OGTT	Classify glucose metabolism

Classification of diabetic association		
Normal values	Impaired fasting glucose, Impaired glucose tolerance	Diabetes mellitus
Fasting<100mg/dl	100-125mg/dl	>126mg/dl
2-hr <140mg/dl	≥140-199mg/dl	≥200mg/dl
HBA1c < 5.7%	5.7-6.4%	≥6.5%

Women with a history of gestational diabetes are also at risk for cardiovascular complications associated with dyslipidaemia, hypertension, and abdominal obesity—the metabolic syndrome. **Akinci and associates** (2009) reported that a fasting glucose level ≥ 100 mg/dl in the index OGTT was an independent predictor of the metabolic syndrome.

In subsequent pregnancies, recurrence was documented in 40 percent of women with gestational diabetes. Lifestyle behavioural changes, including weight control and exercise between pregnancies, likely would prevent gestational diabetes recurrence

(**Kim, 2008**). **Ehrlich and colleagues** (2011) found that the loss of at least two BMI units was associated with a lower risk of gestational diabetes in women who were overweight or obese in the first pregnancy.

NICE guideline for follow up:

Test blood glucose in women who were diagnosed with gestational diabetes to exclude persisting hyperglycaemia before they are transferred to community care.

For women who were diagnosed with gestational diabetes and whose blood glucose levels returned to normal after the birth:

Offer lifestyle advice (including weight control, diet and exercise).

Offer a fasting plasma glucose test 6–13weeks after the birth to exclude diabetes (for practical reasons this might take place at the 6-week postnatal check).

If a fasting plasma glucose test has not been performed by 13weeks, offer a fasting plasma glucose test, or an HbA1c test if a fasting plasma glucose test is not possible, after 13weeks.

Do not routinely offer a 75g 2-hour OGTT.

Offer an annual HbA1c test to women who were diagnosed with gestational diabetes who have a negative postnatal test for diabetes.

Then patients can be divided into following groups:

A) Advise women with a fasting plasma glucose level below 6.0mmol/litre (108mg/dl) that:

-they have a low probability of having diabetes at present

-they should continue to follow the lifestyle advice (including weight control, diet and exercise) given after the birth

-they will need an annual test to check that their blood glucose levels are normal.

-they have a moderate risk of developing type2 diabetes, and offer them advice and guidance in line with the NICE guideline.

B) Advice the women with a fasting plasma glucose level between 6.0 and 6.9mmol/litre (108 to 124mg/dl) that:

-they are at high risk of developing type2 diabetes, and offer them advice, guidance and interventions in line with the NICE guideline on preventing type 2 diabetes.

Advice the women with fasting plasma glucose level of 7.0mmol/litre or above (126mg/dl): that they are likely to have type2 diabetes, and offer them a diagnostic test to confirm diabetes.

For women having an HbA1c test as the postnatal test:

Advice the women with an HbA1c level below 39mmol/l (5.7%) that:

> They have a low probability of having diabetes at present

> They should continue to follow the lifestyle advice (including weight control, diet and exercise) given after the birth

> They will need an annual test to check that their blood glucose levels are normal

> They have a moderate risk of developing type2 diabetes, and offer them advice and guidance in line with the NICE guideline on preventing type 2-diabetes.

Advice the women with an HbA1c level between 39 and 47mmol/l (5.7% and 6.4%) that: they are at high risk of developing type2 diabetes, and offer them advice, guidance and interventions in line with the NICE guideline on preventing.

Advise women with an HbA1c level of 48mmol/l (6.5%) or above that: they have type2 diabetes and refer them for further care.

Offer an annual HbA1c test to women who were diagnosed with gestational diabetes who have a negative postnatal test for diabetes.

Offer women who were diagnosed with gestational diabetes early self-monitoring of blood glucose or an OGTT in future pregnancies. Offer a subsequent OGTT if the first OGTT results in early pregnancy are normal.

Women who have been diagnosed with gestational diabetes should discontinue blood glucose-lowering therapy immediately after birth.

Women with pre-existing type2 diabetes who are breastfeeding can resume or continue to take metformin [4] and glibenclamide [7] immediately after birth, but should avoid other oral blood glucose-lowering agents while breastfeeding.

Women with diabetes who are breastfeeding should continue to avoid any medicines for the treatment of diabetes complications that were discontinued for safety reasons in the preconception period.

Contraception: Low-dose hormonal contraceptives may be used safely by women with recent gestational diabetes. The rate of subsequent diabetes in oral contraceptive users is not significantly different from that in those who did not use hormonal contraception (**Kerlan**, 2010). Importantly, comorbid obesity, hypertension, or dyslipidaemia should direct the choice for contraception toward a method without potential cardiovascular consequences. In these instances, the intrauterine device is a good alternative.

Prevention of type 2 diabetes mellitus:

Type 2 diabetes is diagnosed in adults who are not pregnant by a **glycosylated haemoglobin (HbA$_{1c}$) level of 6.5% (48 mmol/mol) or above.**

A type 2 diabetes diagnosis can also be made by:

1) Random venous plasma glucose concentration the same or greater than 11.1 mmol/l; or
2) Fasting venous plasma glucose concentration the same or greater than 7.0 mmol/l; or
3) 2-hour venous plasma glucose concentration the same or greater than 11.1 mmol/l 2 hours after 75 g anhydrous glucose in an oral glucose tolerance test (OGTT).

Individual risk factors for type 2 diabetes include:

1) Weight (a body mass index [BMI] of 25kg/m$_2$ or more)
2) A large waist circumference (more than 80 cm or 31.5 inches in women and 94 cm or 37 inches in men)
3) Low physical activity levels
4) A family history of type 2 diabetes,
5) History of gestational diabetes
6) Age (being older than 40 or older than 25 for some black and minority ethnic groups).

overweight or obese: is the main contributing factor for type 2 diabetes. In addition, having a large waist circumference increases the risk of developing type 2 diabetes:

1) Men are at high risk if they have a waist circumference of 94–102 cm (37–40 inches). They are at very high risk if it is more than 102 cm.
2) Women are at high risk if they have a waist circumference of 80–88 cm (31.5–35 inches). They are at very high risk if it is more than 88 cm.

Classification	BMI (kg/m$_2$)
Healthy weight	18.5–24.9
Overweight	25–29.9
Obesity I	30–34.9
Obesity II	35–39.9
Obesity III	40 or more

Following guidelines are given by NICE for weight control and prevention of type 2 diabetes.

- Base meals on starchy foods such as potatoes, bread, rice and pasta, choosing wholegrain where possible.
- Eat fibre-rich foods such as oats, beans, peas, lentils, grains, seeds, fruit, vegetables, wholegrain bread and brown rice and pasta.
- Eat at least five portions of a variety of fruit and vegetables each day, in place of foods higher in fat and calories.
- Adopt a low-fat diet.
- Avoid increasing fat or calorie intake
- Consume as little as possible of fried food; drinks and confectionery high in added sugars (such as cakes, pastries and sugar-sweetened drinks); and other food high in fat and sugar (such as some take-away and fast foods).
- Minimise calorie intake from alcohol
- Watch the portion size of meals and snacks, and how often they are eating throughout the day
- Eat breakfast
- Make activities they enjoy, such as walking, cycling, swimming, aerobics and gardening, a routine part of life and build other activity into their daily routine – for example, by taking the
  stairs instead of the lift or taking a walk at lunchtime
- Expect people to lose no more than 0.5–1 kg (1–2 lb) a week.
- To achieve general health benefits: accumulate at least 30 minutes of at least moderate intensity physical activity on 5 or more days of the week.

- To lose weight: most people may need to do 45–60 minutes of moderate-intensity activity a day, particularly if they do not reduce their energy intake.
- People who have been obese and have lost weight may need to do 60–90 minutes of activity a day to avoid regaining weight.

Target while doing above changes should be:

Risk of individuals developing type 2 diabetes is reduced if they achieve one or more of the following:

- Reduce their weight by more than 5%
- Keep their fat intake below 30% of energy intake
- Keep their saturated-fat intake below 10% of energy intake
- Eat 15 g/1000 kcal of fibre or more
- Are physically active for at least 4 hours per week.

www.ingramcontent.com/pod-product-compliance
Lightning Source LLC
Chambersburg PA
CBHW080614180526
45168CB00007B/2907